DENTISTRY

BEYOND THE CLASSROOM

What They Don't Teach You in School
And How to Set Your Business Up for Success

By Theresa Jacks

ISBN | 9780578233451

Imprint | 9780578233451

Bio

Getting to Know Me

My name is Theresa Jacks, and I want to share my story and success with you. I grew up in Calvert County, Maryland in a three-bedroom house on thirty acres of land. I had a few farm animals, a garden in the backyard, and three siblings. We were expected to be home when the street lights came on at six p.m. to spend time with the family and—how could I forget—do our chores. My mother allowed us to be who we were. She treated us fairly and never told us we couldn't achieve our goals in life.

Every Saturday and Sunday, my mother (who did not drive) would fix a ride for us to go to Grandma's house. There were always so many family members around, laughing, cooking, joking, and playing cards while the kids played outside all day. If you needed a meal, you were at the right house. My family taught me the importance of helping others, spending quality time with loved ones, and creating memories. I thank them for that every day, both in my career and with my own family.

However, the country life kept us all very sheltered. While I knew there had to be more to life, I didn't know what—and neither, it seemed, did my mother. In the summer, she worked with my aunts and uncles in the tobacco field to buy us school clothes. As I got older I realized that if my mother had been exposed to the right education and support system, who knows who she would have become? We were too busy living in our small bubble, not exposing our minds to bigger things.

Well, I was going to change that.

I always knew that I would have a career helping others, but was not sure what I wanted to do. Honestly, I wasn't aware of all the jobs that were available. When I was in school, they told us about government jobs and the military. Neither of those struck me as something I wanted to do, so right out of high school I started a career as a cosmetologist. After two years I decided to become a home health aide instead, and after three years of that, I decided to change careers again. Knowing that I still wanted to help people, I began to search the local newspaper. That's when I happened across a job posting for an office manager position at a dental office. I was confident I could do the job.

I applied and got hired the same day.

Three years after I began working at this office, the doctor decided to sell the practice to a corporation so she could retire. She wanted to make sure the team/family she had worked with for years was taken care of. Words can't describe how we all felt.

She allowed us to research the companies she was looking at. Once she decided on the company, she closed the office for a half day and discussed with the team why she picked the company and what they had to offer us. Any questions we had, she addressed, and the ones she did not have answers to, she took notes on and got back to us later. What a blessing to know that the doctor we supported all these years really cared about her team!

We supported her all the way up until the time she left to pursue her dreams. One year after we became affiliated with the new company, I was offered the opportunity to take management classes. This would involve traveling one week a month for six months to focus and grow myself. What an amazing experience and opportunity.

I learned so much—like how you have to build yourself first before you can help others, and how you need to understand yourself and why you think and act the way you do.

In those classes, I realized that I was always focusing on the "how to" of the job, making sure I understood every system and how that system affected the dental practice as a whole, along with techniques on how to improve areas of the business by using metrics. I also realized that my mother never taught me the word failure. I only knew that in order to get results, you need to do things over and over again, trying different methods until it works. Because of this built-in mindset, I am able to get results with everything I put my mind to.

However, there is more to a company than its systems and business techniques. Getting to know your consultant, for instance, is very important. You wouldn't hire a dental partner in your practice without getting to know them well. Hiring the wrong person for your dental-consultant needs is just as bad as hiring an employee that is not a fit for your office.

When I first started out as an office manager, I quickly learned dealing with people can be challenging, so I avoided the people relationships. I looked at the numbers daily and, if I did not see the results I wanted, I stepped in to do the job myself. I was not holding team members accountable because my belief was that no one could do it better or faster than I could. Only I knew how to get the results.

What I didn't realize was that I was not growing anyone, because I didn't train them on how I got my results. Of course I was the only one who could do it right—I never bothered to teach anyone else how to do it!

So I worked on (what I now know to be called) my "doers" dilemma and started training and empowering my team members to do the tasks I had to let go of. It was so hard to give up control of what had become my baby, but in the end, the company ran smoother and better without my constant eye on every detail.

I knew that I had a gift for closing cases, but what I didn't know at the time was that I knew how to read people. I could quickly determine which patients wanted a lot of information, who just wanted to know the fees, and who I needed to spend more time with, getting to know them and letting them know they needed to take care of themselves so that they could continue to take care of their loved ones. Today, I realize that I was instinctually working with the deciphering of DISC personality traits. After my classes, I was able to teach this skill to everyone in the business. Soon, we all had that "gift."

What changed my life was when I started working on building relationships—first with the doctor, so the team could see us as business partners. Once that was established, I worked on my relationships with the team. Then it was much easier for me to implement change and create effective systems. I realized that I was getting results at a much faster rate. I was inspiring motivation and I led by example. I held team members accountable, I had conversations with them in the moments when things weren't going right, and I did all this by asking questions, not assuming. In the process of doing this, I have built some very long-lasting relationships with people who have told me how inspiring I am.

In this book, I hope to share what I have learned over my years of education, experience, and growth in the dental business, so your dental business can blossom as well!

Table of Contents

CHAPTER 1:	# Building relationships with your patients
	Relationship building is key. The initial contact starts when the patient makes the first phone call to your office. Make sure you hire the right person to be on the phone for this call.

Once the patient comes into your office, having a great patient intake form will allow you to gather some important information.

Top five questions to ask on the intake form:

1. What brought you to our office?

2. Who, if anyone, referred you?

3. Any concerns—pain or swelling, broken teeth/tooth, sensitivity to temperature or sweets?

4. Any past experiences with previous dentists you want to share? What did you like or dislike?

    (This question will give you a guide on how to treat the patient when they come into the office. If they disliked waiting for too long at their last place, for example, make sure you seat them in a timely manner.) |

5. Can I have your insurance information?

A great website to use for this form is www.patientintakechecklistfordentalclinic.com, which will allow you to customize the form to your liking.

If possible, verify the new patient's insurance before they walk into the office. Use this website to get a free copy of an insurance verification form: www.freedentalinsuranceverificationform.com.

Once your new patient has arrived in the office, make sure you address their chief concerns. Put the treatment prescribed on the treatment plan as order number one, then put your recommended treatment next. This shows the patient that you are listening to them instead of trying to upsell, or recommending whatever procedure costs more.

There are three types of listening:

1. A "Listen About" Listener is

- not an active participant in the conversation
- mentally fading in and out of focus
- not actually concerned with what the other person is saying

2. A "Listen For" Listener is

- looking only for the opportunity to speak

- analyzing or prejudging content before the other person is finished speaking

3. A "Listen To" Listener is

- involved in and mentally present for the conversation

- reading between the lines

- making clarifying statements

"Listening to" is the truest and most sincere form of listening.

Treatment planning is another important part of the practitioner-patient relationship. Are you giving the patient all of the treatment needed on the first visit? Or are you communicating to the patient they have a lot going on, so you will be focusing on one area at a time? Or are you asking the patients how they want the information, so it's not overwhelming to them?

Remember, building relationships is not about us; it's about them. The moment you make it about you, you are no longer building a relationship.

Quadrant treatment planning (breaking up the treatment plan into smaller chunks) will feel less overwhelming to the patient and will increase your closing rate.

A hypothetical patient experience without quadrant planning:

Ms. Jones walked into a dental office as a new patient. Her chief concern was a broken front tooth. After her dental exam, she was presented with a treatment plan for over $5,000. When she looked at the treatment plan, she only looked at the $5,000 and quickly replied, "I can't afford this. You guys are too expensive." She left the office upset and still with her broken tooth. Later, she went on social media and left a negative review.

A hypothetical patient experience with quadrant planning:

Ms. Jones walked into a dental office as a new patient. Her chief concern was a broken front tooth. After her dental exam she was presented with a treatment plan for $5,000. When she looked at the treatment plan, she noticed it was broken down into two visits. The first visit was for her broken tooth, which she would pay $500 for out of pocket, and on the second visit, she would pay $4,500 for a bridge. Ms. Jones was happy to know that fixing the tooth wouldn't cost as much as she thought. She got started with treatment the same day and made an appointment to come back for the bridge. She left the office very happy. Then she went on social media and raved about the doctor and staff.

Tip: Small talk can also help your patients feel more comfortable in what is usually an uncomfortable setting for them. Here are some sample questions to ask your patients to build rapport:

1. What did you like most about your last dentist?

2. Have you had any big events or good news happen lately?

3. What type of movies do you like, or what was the last movie you saw?

Mastering practitioner-patient communication will directly add value to your patients and your bottom line, allowing your business to grow.

CHAPTER 2:

Closing the case: getting your patients to accept treatment

Presentation is key when outlining treatment plans for your patients.

First, always be confident. Review x-rays and make sure you have all of the information from your hygienist about the patient before you walk into the room. When speaking to patients, make sure you are using words or analogies they can understand. The most important thing a patient needs to know is how much you care about them. If you can master this, your patients will be much happier and more forgiving if you make a mistake.

Second, help your patient see their problem. Educate your patients on what is called PCS:

P: Problem. You need to identify this before you can do anything else.

C: Consequence of not fixing the problem. This interaction is important because it motivates the patient to move forward with treatment. *Do not skip over this step*. It is vital in helping your patients understand what will happen if they decide not to do treatment.

S: Solution. This is the treatment your patient needs. Make sure to give the patient options; however, do not overwhelm them with a lot of information. This will cause a patient to become "paralyzed," and they may feel so overwhelmed they will not be able to make a decision. Try not to use limiting words or phrases, like "It's just a little filling," and stress the urgency of getting the work done sooner to prevent more expensive treatment down the line.

"Nobody cares how much you know until they know how much you care."
—Theodore Roosevelt

Tips for getting your patient to agree to treatment:

1. Always schedule the next appointment while the patient is still in the chair. Patients will then feel like it's a part of their appointment time. If you allow them to walk up to the front desk to schedule, patients will feel it is less urgent and say things like, "I need to check with my husband/wife," or "I need to check my calendar." They are ready to get out of the office and go back to work or home, so scheduling becomes an inconvenience. Remember, it is the job of the dentist and dental assistant to keep the schedule full, and allowing patients to schedule once they leave the chair often results in a lost opportunity.

2. If the patient does not schedule while they are in the office, walk back into the room once your treatment coordinator is finished and let the patient know that you are here whenever they need you if they have any more questions. This will allow the patient to feel important and helps them believe that you care about them.

Closing the case and getting your patients to agree to treatment builds your reputation and potential for growth. Developing and implementing this process appropriately will allow your business to thrive.

CHAPTER 3:	# Building a strong relationship with your hygienists

Making sure your hygienists are following your expectations is important for the longevity of your business. It is also important they feel satisfied in their work.

It's a good idea to have weekly or monthly meetings to discuss philosophy of care and your expectations. You want to make sure your whole team is on the same page.

Topics to ensure your hygienists are in agreement on may include the following:

Fluoride:

- Reduces risk of new decay.
- Reduces sensitivity.
- Explain to patients that fluoride protects their teeth.

Sealants:

- Take photos and use these to increase the level of urgency.
- There is a 95% chance of eventually experiencing caries in pits and fissures in posterior teeth if a sealant is not placed.
- Recommended on all permanent posterior teeth.

Desensitizers:

- Can last up to three years, and you can touch up in between.

- About 80% of adults suffer from sensitive teeth.

- Try it out on the patient's most sensitive tooth. If it doesn't work, they don't need to pay for it.

Oral Cancer Screening (VELscope):

- In the United States, one person dies from oral cancer every hour.

- About 90% of all oral cancer is curable if caught early.

- The American Cancer Society recommends all adults eighteen years and older get screened once a year.

Same-Day Treatment:

- Remind your hygienists, if possible, to ask patients, "Would you like to get this taken care of today?" The patient may have to wait for an hour or so, but taking care of a procedure on the same day is both beneficial to your business and will more likely result in your patient being satisfied and willing to accept treatment.

- Let the doctor and team know ASAP if the patient accepts same-day treatment so the room can be set up.

Canceled Appointments:

- Remember that every broken or canceled appointment is an opportunity to schedule another patient.

Tips: It's also important to develop good rapport with your hygienists. Here are some sample conversation topics:

1. What is going well?

2. What opportunities do you have to improve? Or to grow in your career?

3. Is there anything I can help you with?

Always give positive feedback first, then ask permission to share opportunities for improvement. Hold your hygienists accountable by making sure they are following your expectations through weekly one-on-one meetings as well as group meetings. Make sure you are looking out for their needs as well as your business needs to foster growth and profit.

CHAPTER 4:	# Are you paying for yourself?

This is a question that many dentists don't think about.

Whatever you decide to pay yourself and your hygienists weekly, multiply that by four (the number of weeks in a month). This is how much you and your hygienists should aim to bring in monthly.

Add the numbers for each of your hygienists and yourself to get the monthly production goal for the office.

You should be collecting 98–100% of this total monthly goal at the bare minimum.

It's up to you to create an environment where achieving this is possible. Pay careful attention to these five cornerstones:

1. Growth in leadership
2. Accountability for yourself and others
3. Inspiration (where your hygienists find satisfaction in their work for themselves, not just for you)
4. Creating or leading change
5. Overall results

Create an environment where people don't want to disappoint you. Have morning huddles to discuss tasks for the day and outstanding treatment. Also, as mentioned in Chapter 3, hold monthly meetings to discuss broader team issues and goals. As the leader, it is your job to inspire and hold your staff accountable as well as listen to their concerns and implement changes. People don't leave companies; they leave managers. Pay attention to how well you are operating your business by calculating the monthly production numbers and measuring against your goal. Then address changes in your leadership as needed.

"It's never wrong to do the right thing."
—Mark Twain

Tip: This formula is only used to ensure that, at the bare minimum, you are paying for yourself. In order to run a successful business and be able to pay bills, etc., your monthly goal should be much higher.

Overall, remember that you should be measuring your success as the leader of your practice and taking responsibility for meeting your monthly goal.

CHAPTER 5:	# Hiring the right team members
	Your team members are a direct reflection of you. When you are opening up a new business and want to attract customers, you are going to need a rock-star front desk and office manager. (Or a front desk manager and a dental consultant, which is also a possibility.)
	Things to look for in the hiring process:
	First of all, remember that this process is not meant to hurt anyone; it is used to find the best candidate for your business. It doesn't matter how much education is on the resume—if the person is not a right fit for your business, you are going to lose money if you hire them. You can teach someone how to do procedures, but you can't teach personality or work ethic.
	Second, you need to invest in your team members. There is no such thing as the perfect hire, so be willing to teach and train someone to align with your philosophies and practice. If you can be open to understanding this, you will hire people who will stay with you throughout the duration of your career. These candidates tend to be loyal and flexible, and they will be so grateful that you invested in them.

Third, don't be afraid to hire someone with experience. They could be a great asset to your business, especially if you need someone to help guide the day-to-day operations. Someone who already knows how to run an office, how to hire people, and is familiar with the software you are using would typically be a great fit for an office manager.

Things to pay attention to during the interview process:

1. How long did it take them to get back to you after you left the first voicemail? The answer to this question will tell you if this person is punctual and reliable. Keep in mind, though, they may be at work and unable to answer or return your call. Take notes on every contact with the candidates so you can determine any possible issues.

2. Make sure you ask: "Why are you leaving your current job?" If the candidate says, "Because it's too far away from home," look at the resume and ask how long of a commute the other jobs were. Then ask follow-up questions like, "I see you have been traveling for years, why is it important for you to be close to home now?" You would be surprised by the information that can come out of this question—

things you might not have learned if you had just allowed them to answer the question and you moved on to the next question.

3. Ask situational questions to see how they think. Example: You have two patients scheduled at 2 p.m. The first patient is running late, so you took the other 2 p.m. patient back. While you were doing that, an emergency patient walked in at the same time your 2 p.m. patient who is running late walked in. Who do you take back first? These questions are great because there may not be a clear right or wrong answer. You want to see how this person would handle this kind of situation, and it's the perfect time to let them know how you expect the patient flow to be handled in your office.

4. Have they moved around a lot from job to job? Find out why and ask how the process was for them from one job to the other: How long did it take? Why do you think it took as long as it did? You want to see if they blame others, make up excuses, or take responsibility without blame. The candidates who blame others or have an excuse for everything are not going to be a good fit for your business. You need

people who take responsibility. These candidates are usually at work when they are scheduled to be at work, and they don't take off much.

5. Make sure you are hiring someone who can get along with your current team members. This is huge. If, for example, you have a lot of straightforward, strong personalities in the office, it would not be a good fit to hire someone who is quiet and shy, as they might feel like they are being attacked in conversations with straightforward, strong personalities. Before you begin the hiring process, learn DISC personality types to help you with selecting the right members for your team. Go to www.discinsights.com for more information. This will help you in a lot of other communication areas as well. If you can master this, the benefit will be greater than you can imagine—in the office, and in everyday life.

6. I can't express the importance of making sure your existing team is involved in the hiring process of new members. They may see things you don't. Alternatively, the candidate may feel more comfortable asking questions or sharing things with a team member that they did not feel

comfortable discussing with you. My interviews usually take one hour to one and a half hours. On the same day as the interview, I usually ask if the candidate can stay for thirty minutes to shadow the team (I ask this the day I set up the interview, allowing two hours. As you get better at interviewing, this process may only take one hour). The applicant will shadow whatever role they are looking to fill (except for the position of hygienist, in which case the applicant will shadow the doctor and dental assistant).

Tips for interviewing:

1. Remember this process is not intended to judge anyone; this is about asking probing questions to discover any red flags.

2. The method of asking questions one by one and getting them to share—following instead of leading the discussion—is called Sherlocking. Ask clarifying questions about what they shared in hopes that they will share more. This method should always leave the person feeling respected and heard. It is information gathering, not problem solving.

3. Take time to learn DISC with your entire team. Once they can spot

red flags as well as you, the hiring process will be much easier—and it will be fun!

If you can master the interview process, you will hire great people, which will mean happier patients who will come back and refer other patients to you.

CHAPTER 6:

Are you checking your lab bills monthly?

This includes Invisalign bills and all other bills you receive in the office by invoice.

When it comes to paperwork and bills, everyone makes mistakes. By keeping your invoices and matching them to your final monthly bill, you can make sure you are being charged the correct amount. Keeping a file for invoices monthly is a great idea.

Assign this job to a dental assistant to free up more of your own time. It is also important to get your dental assistant involved in this process because he/she is going to be vital in helping you save money as he/she becomes more aware of the financial side of the business.

Tip: You can never be too careful when it comes to checking the bills. Paying careful attention to the numbers will ensure your business is not losing money when it shouldn't be.

CHAPTER 7:	# Are you using affordable dental supplies?

Dental supplies can cost a fortune. This is an area where you should be flexible about brands—ask for free samples or give other brands a try, and if they don't work for you, no problem. Think about it like this: How many products do you know of that have a generic brand? Same ingredients, but different brand names? Why pay more if you don't have to? Pick and choose the things you can save on; however, the more flexible you can be in this area, the more you will bring to your bottom line. In no way should you compromise your patient care to save money, but if the product is the same, why pay more?

Tip: Just because you are not paying top dollar for a product does not always mean it's of lower quality. When choosing a dental assistant to be in charge of ordering, find out who likes to save money and find deals. This is your ideal person to be in charge of ordering supplies.

Be open to trying different products and selecting those that are both beneficial to your patients and your business.

CHAPTER 8:

Are you collecting at 98–100% of your monthly production?

Keep an eye on this area daily. Make sure your front desk team is collecting co-payments the same day. If not, find out what the barriers are. Staying on top of collections is the best way to keep money flowing into the office. Make sure you are having weekly meetings to discuss how much you did in production versus how much you collected. You don't want to wait until the end of the month to notice that you did not collect enough money to cover your overhead costs, causing you to fall behind in the negative.

How does this happen, you ask? Well, it all starts from the new patient phone call.

Things to verify:

1. Did you get the correct insurance information? The correct policy-holder's name, date of birth, ID number, and insurance contact number to verify benefits? Verification of benefits should be done the day before your patient arrives at the office so everything runs smoothly during their appointment.

2. Did you enter the insurance information correctly in the system? Make sure you are scanning the new patient registration form, a valid ID, and the front and back of the insurance card. You will need this information to verify correct entry into the system.

3. Did you call the insurance company to get a full breakdown along with deductibles, yearly max, waiting clauses, missing tooth clauses, downgrades, pay on seat or prep date, frequency, and limitations? What fee schedule should you use along with the payor ID number? If you are doing orthodontic work, make sure you are verifying benefits for the codes you are using, along with how often they pay. This is important to know because some insurance companies pay automatically, while others require you to send in a claim every three months. For SRP, are all four quadrants covered the same day? What is the frequency, and is FMD covered? When is the benefit year and night guard coverage—and is it for bruxism only? Are composites downgraded? Is there sealant coverage? What teeth numbers? How often can it be done? What is the age limit? Any implant

coverage? Limitations on x-rays fmx and bwx's? Fluoride coverage?

4. Did you enter the correct percentage into the system, along with the patient's remaining available max? A great way to check this is to look at the EOB form when it comes back to the insurance company, then look at the patient's treatment plan that they signed before getting treatment done. Did you estimate the correct co-pay? If not, take a look at the suggestions above and see where your area of opportunity is. Discuss this weekly in your business meeting with your office manager.

5. When co-payments are not being collected the day of treatment, make sure the front desk is putting detailed notes in the patient's file. Verify this daily.

Tips:

1. If you plan to give discounts, make sure you are offering discounts to everyone. Otherwise, this could cause many issues. For example: "My neighbor and I are both patients at your office. We both have Delta Dental, and we both had crowns done on the same day. In a conversation with my neighbor, I found out she was given $100 off her crown, but I paid full price." This kind of practice

can be viewed as discrimination or favoritism, since both patients had the same procedure and insurance (which already gave them a discount because you were an in-network provider). Be careful. You don't know who knows each other outside of your office.

2. If you plan to give a senior discount or a discount to patients without insurance, remember to give this discount equally to those meeting the criteria.

3. Another very important tip regarding this subject is if your patient has insurance that you are in network with and you give that patient a discount, you must put that on the claim form in the unusual remarks section.

Being consistent with patient billing is critical to your business growth. Make sure to collect the appropriate information at the start and be fair when giving discounts.

CHAPTER 9:

Are your insurance aging reports and patient aging reports getting completed before the end of the month?

Completing the insurance aging and patient aging reports by the 15th of every month gives patients and insurance companies from then until the end of the month to send in payments.

To stay on track:

1. Print both reports on the first of the month.

2. Work on the accounts daily. Call patients to collect balances, call insurance companies to follow up on claims that are over thirty days old with no payment, etc.

Remember: Make sure you are collecting 98–100% of your average monthly production as you look at these reports.

CHAPTER 10:	# Putting systems in place
	The biggest challenge in the dental office can be creating systems for your front desk. It is very important that everyone answering the phones and greeting patients are all on the same page when it comes to communication and office policies.

Over my twenty-five-year career, I've learned a lot from private practices and corporate dentistry. I've created systems and created my own checklists that I've used to hold my teams accountable.

I've attached my expectation forms below. Keep in mind that you will have to adjust these forms to fit your office. |

Check-In Desk

Greet Patients

Introduce yourself, ask if any information has changed, and verify insurance.

Mark the patient as present and announce arrival.

Have the patient fill out and sign medical history forms over three years old.

Update address, phone numbers, email accounts, and INS information upon check-in.

DO NOT FORGET TO UPDATE IN DENTRIX

Make sure all NEW patients signed the registration form, and a referral source is attached in the Family File.

Make sure we scan a copy of their driver's license and insurance card in the patient's file.

Attach the insurance ASAP.

Account Aging Reports/ Insurance Aging Reports

Review the last statement and guarantor balance.

Any patients with a guarantor balance who did not receive a statement during the last bulk mailing will be sent a statement. Mail today.

Verify with each insurance company that the current claim is/is not on file. We will resend and check the re-sent box.

Take detailed notes on who you talked to and what you sent with your initials.

Do 50Q insurance verification WITHIN TWENTY-FOUR HOURS. On Friday, do Saturday and Monday.

#1 Rock (Schedule) Fill Schedule

Work Unscheduled Treatment, ASAP, Broken Appts, New Patient list, Overdue Recall.

Fill the schedule for the next day, before you leave!

Note how many calls were made from each list and how many patients were scheduled to add to your personal accountability goals.

Fill out the daily checklist and include a copy with an end-of-day packet.

Confirmation calls done by 10 a.m. for appointments that are two days out. Write on the schedule who confirmed and who didn't.

End of Day

Run insurance reports and correct.

Check for insurance not processed.

Check for secondary insurances not sent.

Check for procedures not attached to claims.

Pull SWOTs for the next day and ensure 50Q verifications are done. Call patients and get the information if needed.

Miscellaneous

Complete weekly RGB report due to manager by close of business day Friday.

Check smile reminders.

Update doctor's calendar daily.

Update monthly balancing report daily.

MONTHLY TIMETABLE

15th of the month—insurance aging report completed.

15th of the month—statements sent.

30th of the month—collection calls made on all accounts over 30 days old without payment. Prepare accounts for collections.

Chart prep. Make sure there is a G-Note on all of the accounts with a balance. Check to see if we have a signed Tx plan on file for the work being done today and next visit. (Tx plan must be signed within 30 days.)

Before you present treatment plans, always look at the breakdown to ensure there are not any waiting periods, missing tooth clauses, or age limits!!!! Check to see if fillings on molars are downgraded!!!! (VERY IMPORTANT)

	2 on 1 transfer to the second shift
	How many calls did you make today?
	How many calls did you complete successfully?
	Signature:
	Date:

Check-Out Desk

Opening Duties

Print morning huddle form and email to your PA daily.

Check emails. Respond to emails sent to the office and copy your PA.

Sign into PSR Portals.

Start filling holes in the schedule today and follow up with your doctor.

50Q insurance verification.

Assure all items are ready for the morning huddle.

Check-Out

Call patients who are not confirmed for today.

Introduce yourself and ask how their appointment went. Make sure the next two appointments have been scheduled.

Present treatment plan in TREATMENT ROOM or CONSULT ROOM, not at the front desk.

Make appointments for operative and hygiene procedures (prior to collecting the money due).

Make sure all procedures are entered correctly under the correct provider.

Make sure we are charging out the correct fees, if patient had the $59 mailer.

Attach appropriate files to claim (x-rays and/or period charting).

Collect for the "FAMILY BALANCE," not just today's procedures. (Example: Fee is $295; however, they have an outstanding balance that totals $483. Instead of explaining everything, say, "Ms. Smith, your balance is $483 for today." Most will not ask anything else. Don't go into details unless you have to.)

Print walkout statement and verify that all family members have appointments.

DON'T LET ANYONE LEAVE WITHOUT AN APPOINTMENT!!! YOU CAN DO IT WITH THE RIGHT STRATEGY!

"Ms. Smith, I understand you need to check your schedule; however, the doctor's schedule is really full. He/she will need a bit of time for this appointment and would like you to get in ASAP before any problems with that tooth arise. I would feel safer if we scheduled you now, and then if that date/time doesn't work, we can always reschedule, as long as you promise you will call me as soon as you can."

Ask the patient for a referral, go over current specials (bleaching, Invisalign, etc.).

Handle account audits and patient inquiries.

Send in any refund requests.

OM Development Plan

Communication, on all levels, is a must.

- Before you act, communicate for alignment.
- When looking to communicate or vent, always communicate up and only discuss the issues with the person(s) involved.
- Contact your doctor as needed to discuss current events.
- Ask for help when needed and accept it when offered.
- Send your recaps within twenty-four hours. This helps everyone see the value you are adding in your role.

Acting in line with the fundamentals and core values of the company is the only way to make your dental practice successful.

- If something is out of line, bring it to the doctor's attention.
- Practice expense control: salary under 20%, right sized team, limited OT, professional supplies under 4.5%, using preferred products list. Labs under 4.5%, using preferred labs.
- Development of monthly and quarterly action plans to consistently move the practice forward in support of the doctor's goals.

Your role is demanding and rewarding. You are a partner to your doctor(s).

- Be confident.
- Be accountable and stay true to your top ten professional goals and the goals of your doctor(s).

Uphold the level of accountability needed to self, team, doctor(s), and patient in meeting deadlines, keeping your word, meeting individual needs, and following through.

- Once commitments are made, follow-through is expected to be completed in a timely and efficient manner. Always underpromise and overdeliver!

- Reports: Hold yourself and your team accountable to reporting on time. The earlier, the better, especially with the following:

  - BA calendar

  - A/R checklist

  - Recare checklist

  - Credit balance

  - Chart audits

Avoid crisis management:

- Recognize that having crucial conversations ahead of time—when handled professionally, quickly, and effectively—will end in a win-win result and actually save you time in the long run.

- When communicating, adjust to the personality of the person you are speaking to using DISC.

- Always remember to prioritize tasks according to the level of danger involved.

- Be a part of the solution rather than adding fuel to the fire by not being well prepared for conversations.

- Document, document, document!

- Bring up any "red flags" and action items as well as proposed solutions when you are uncertain.

Relationships: Partnering with your doctor(s) in all things is the number-one key to success.

- The importance of building and maintaining a positive relationship and work environment with your doctors and each of your team members creates the loyalty and teamwork needed to achieve the goals of the doctor, the practice, and the team members themselves.

- Spend time before and after the morning huddle to discuss what the team members want to accomplish each day.

Importance of numbers and results:

1. Ask yourself daily:

   - "How can I make a difference today?"

   - "Am I holding the team accountable by providing feedback?"

2. Review the numbers daily, weekly, and monthly. Partner with the doctor(s) to provide support in achieving their goals for the practice and team.

3. Focus on the key metrics that are below a thriving level or trending down.

   - Recare 90%

   - DSO thirty days

   - % to budget

   - Collections to production 94%

4. Focus on Lifetime Care and the goals of the doctor(s) for the practice.

   - New patient flow.

   - Daily conversions.

   - Hygiene department support: production per hour and RVU efficiency.

Change is going to happen.

- It is inevitable, so view it as a challenge—not an inconvenience.
- Grow from the challenges.
- Encourage others to adapt through your reactions to change.

Continuing education:

- Read at least one book per month on anything

Technical expectations of a leader:

- *Be a coach, not a cheerleader.*
- *Live in the present and live with passion.*
- *Be a long-term thinker.*
- *Be a risk-taker—mistakes are opportunities to learn. As long as your actions are connected with the company mission and vision (and your doctor(s) support you), all will be fine.*
- *Be independent and also interdependent. Know your resources and use them!*
- *Avoid fault-finding. Address concerns in the moment and seek solutions.*
- *Be a thermostat (solution-focused, adjustable, and adaptable) not a thermometer (merely providing information).*
- *Get comfortable with upsets. Being a leader, a coach, or even a parent requires dealing with the occasional upset as we guide and teach.*
- *Inspire. Lead well, and they will follow.*
- *Make work fun. Be sure all doctors and team members want to come to work.*

- *Maintain a positive balance in everyone's emotional bank account. Make more deposits (positive feedback and recognition) than withdrawals (reprimand and negative feedback). If this is hard, maybe you're overspending!*

- *Make a difference every day.*

- **And have fun!!!!**

Dental Assistant Daily Check-Off List

DATE: _____

DA NAME:_____

ROOM NUMBERS _____

Preparing rooms before your shift:

____ Fill patient bibs, barrier tape, headrest covers, handle covers.

____ Prepare suction tips and air/water tips.

____ Fill water bottles (both on the chair and assistant table).

____ Fill sundries (cotton rolls, 2x2 gauze, micro brushes, etc.).

____ Fill triple trays of all sizes.

____ Fill impression materials and tips (heavy body, light body, and bite registration).

____ Fill gloves and masks (both on the doctor's side and the assistant's side).

____ Fill anesthetic (all types) and needles (all types).

____ Fill etch, bond, desensitizer, vitrebond, IRM, condensable composite in all shades, flowable in all shades, and polishing paste.

____ Stock mixing pads, fujicem/relyx cement (and tips), core buildup material (and tips), temp crown material (and tips), try-in paste (and tips), and tempbond clear (and tips).

____ Handheld mirror is in the room and clean.

____ Put clean glasses in the room.

____ Check the floors for debris. Sweep and mop as needed. (Always mop the last day of the week.)

___ Counters are wiped and clean.

___ Pens and clipboards present.

___ Cavicide gauze stocked.

___ Clean cabinet doors and counters with Lysol.

___ Update storage inventory.

___ Check tomorrow's lab cases. (Make sure all are ready; otherwise, reschedule patient.)

___ Add paper towels to the dispenser.

___ Sign autoclave and disinfection logs.

___ Suction/air valves turned off (if end of day).

DA Signature_____

Manager Signature _____

Hygiene Expectations

1. Patients seated at appropriate time—no later than ten minutes after forms are complete.

2. Make a conscious effort to communicate and build a relationship with the patient before you ever look in their mouth. This will especially help anxious patients.

3. Ask about previous dental experiences.

4. Take digital photo of their smile, as well as intraoral photos of potential restorative needs. Project them onto TV to discuss with the patient as part of preheat.

5. FMS (full mouth series) and pano for new patients twenty-one years old and over.

    i.   4 BWX and pano for NPs children ages twelve to twenty.

    ii. 2 BWX and pano for children ages six (possibly younger) to twelve.

6. Documentation and discussion of perio charting scores.

7. Documentation of diagnosis and reasoning in clinical chart.

8. Proper reflection in chart of preexisting conditions.

9. Preheat patients on anticipated treatment.

10. Proper transfer with either hygienist or assistant. (This needs to be more clear than saying, "Mrs. Jones is feeling good today and has good oral hygiene.")

11. Going over:

    i.   Periodontal disease and reasons for SRP "normal cleaning/prophy."

   ii. VELscope for all new patients during comprehensive exam, then annually, especially for those with a tobacco habit.

12.   Review schedule and make two-week calls.

Signature: Date:

www.ingramcontent.com/pod-product-compliance
Lightning Source LLC
Chambersburg PA
CBHW061449180526
45170CB00004B/1626